Yoga Basics for Beginners
A Simple Guide to Yoga for
Beginners for Health, Fitness and
Happiness

Ntathu Allen

Editor

Marjorie Kramer

Marjorie.Kramer@gmail.com

YOGA BASICS FOR BEGINNERS

A Simple Guide To Yoga For Beginners For Health, Fitness And Happiness

Ntathu Allen

Table of Contents

Get Even More

Just to say "Thank You" for purchasing this book,
I WANT TO GIVE YOU A GIFT

100% Absolutely FREE

Meditation For Beginners

Learn How To Effectively Meditate In Comfort From Your Own Home! ... In 5-Minutes A Day

http://freedownload5-minuteguidedmeditation.gr8.com/

Discover Other Titles by Ntathu Allen

Below you'll find some of my other books that are popular on Amazon and Kindle. Simply click on the links below to check them out. Alternatively, you can visit my author page on Amazon to see other work done by me.

Back Care – Yoga Exercises for Lower Back Care at Work: Reduce Stress, Boost Energy and Improve Posture http://amzn.to/1jXOY9r

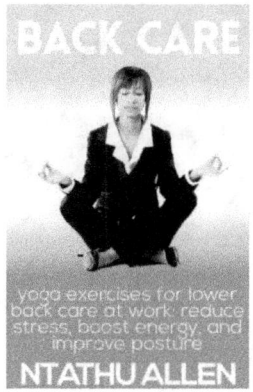

Yoga For Beginners – The Busy Woman's Guide to Easy Yoga Poses and Meditation Techniques to Relieve Stress at Work and Find Peace and Quiet at Home http://amzn.to/1mzNt13

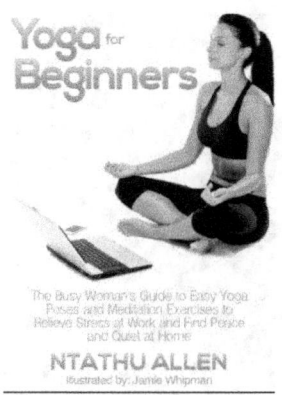

Healing After Loss – Devotional Poems for Healing and Peacehttp://amzn.to/1nQPVQk

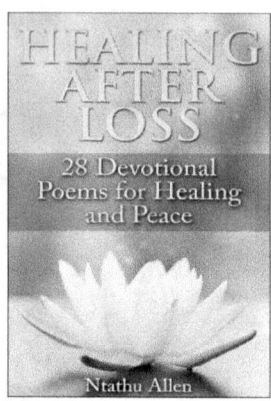

Pray As You Go: Seven Meditation Techniques You Wish You Knew for Healing and Happiness
http://tinyurl.com/l73sodq

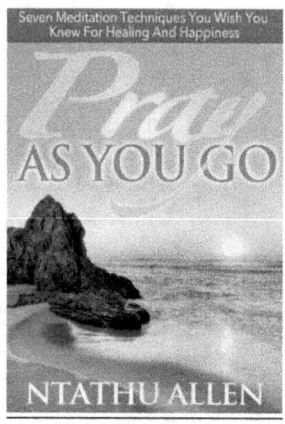

Work Happy: 26 Empowering Tips for Women Entrepreneurs to Stop Stress Now, Supercharge Your Energy and Finally Enjoy Work
http://tinyurl.com/pgb6jkp

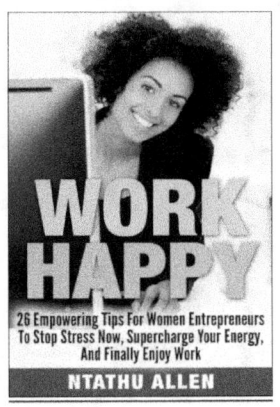

Quick Fix Meditation: The Ultimate Meditation Guide for People Too Busy to Meditate
http://www.amazon.com/dp/B00PE8SYTW

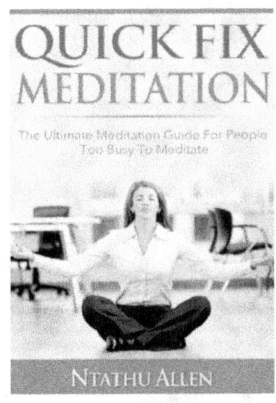

If the links do not work for whatever reason, you can simply search for these titles on the Amazon website to find them

Disclaimer

The aim of this e-Book is to provide general information only and should not be treated as a substitute for the medical advice of your doctor or any other health care professional. The information is intended to help you choose the right style of yoga class for you. It is based on my personal and professional experience of studying and teaching yoga.

The eBook makes no guarantees of success or implied promises. The publisher and author are not responsible or liable for any diagnosis made by a reader based on the contents of this book. Always consult your doctor before starting the exercises in this book and if you are in anyway concerned about your health.

Copyright

As with any form of exercise, please exercise caution, respect and patience for your body. Consult your GP before embarking on any exercise programme. As you practice, be gentle and move slowly into the stretch. Any form of discomfort or strain, please stop and relax.

As you practice the seated **yoga exercises, breathing and meditation exercises in this book,** pay attention to the way you feel and notice any sensations and impressions you feel in your body; your body is a marvelous piece of magic, treat her well and she will serve you well in return.

Remember as you practice to breathe in and gently through your nose and focus your awareness of the part or parts of body where you feel the stretch the most. Be gentle, loving and attentive to what is happening inside your body.

Dedication

To you, gentle reader for your love, trust and re-awakening to the joys and beauty of yoga.

I hope this helps you live a life of vibrant health, fitness and happiness.

Praise From Happy Yoga Students

"I have been attending Ntathu's class for the last six to nine months. I can honestly say it has made a positive change to my life. Overall my strength and flexibility have improved, as well as mentally I feel a lot calmer. Not too long ago, I would worry constantly now I adopt the outlook that things will always work out.

"My initial motivation for taking up yoga was to increase flexibility. As time has gone on, I realize how important learning to breathe properly, plays in calming and energizing the body and mind.

"I am very lucky to have a great teacher in Ntathu. She has such a very calming aura and is very approachable. Attending her class is definitely the highlight of the week for me. I have so much to learn. Hopefully I can motive myself to keep practicing yoga for many years to come." **Michael**

"Dear Ntathu, thank you again for all the time we have spent together and your generosity of spirit! I have learnt a lot from you and gained so much! You inspire me. I wish you so well in all your ventures, your training, business and teaching. May you be blessed by what you give to others in all you do." **Sharon**

"I would recommend yoga to others lead by Ntathu." **Nursery Worker, London**

"I cherish my time with Ntathu. My time with her doing yoga has allowed me to become more aware of myself has provided focus and strength for me to grow and nourishes me spiritually. It is my weekly treat." **Lesley Powls**

Introduction

Yoga helps you live a life of inner peace, happiness and radiant health.

The other day I received a phone call from Mary, a potential yoga student. She was stressed, overworked and exhausted.

Life was getting her down.

In desperation, Mary went to see her Doctor as her migraines were becoming more severe and she struggled to focus at work and sleep at night.

As part of her treatment, Mary's GP suggested Mary "relax more" and "maybe take up yoga or meditation to help her cope better with stress."

As I listened to Mary recall her daily struggle, waking up tired, anxious and clock-watching about getting her children to child care on time; feeling unprepared for her weekly team meetings and the manic rush to pick her children up from child care. I remembered how anxious I used to feel working as a Probation Officer, juggling heavy workloads with a young family.

I was glad Mary was making an effort to tackle her stress.

However, what came next was a shock.

Mary said "looking for a yoga class" was adding to her stress!
Mary moaned that there are so many different styles and types of yoga advertised, that she didn't know where to start or who to trust.

She was not sure what style of yoga would suit her lifestyle and support her desire to learn how to relax and overcome stress. So, I spent about 20 minutes on the phone, listening to Mary share her concerns and answering her questions.
Mary isn't alone.

From my experience of teaching yoga, potential students feel stuck and unsure about yoga. Like Mary, their GP recommends they take up yoga for health reasons or they know friends and work colleagues who practice and feel and look great, yet they are confused and unsure what style of yoga is most suited to their lifestyle and particular health needs.

That's why I wrote this book.

To offer you simple suggestions to ease any concerns and worries you may have about starting yoga. And hopefully encourage you to take the next step and sign-up for a yoga class. If you are a more experienced yogi you will also find the information useful to remind you of the common mistakes and pitfalls you make when you practice and also offer you a brief outline on the more spiritual and philosophical aspects of yoga.

If you feel like Mary, overwhelmed, exhausted and looking for a way out of your current poor health situation, then I pray you will find all your concerns and questions answered in this book,

Stay Blessed and Enjoy Your Yoga Journey

Namaste
Ntathu Allen

About This Book

Feel free to read this book any which way you like. It is a self-help e-book to support you discover how yoga, meditation and your breath can support you feel healthy, happy and more at ease in your body.

Chapter One opens with a general overview and benefits of practicing yoga and in chapter Two we look at the different styles of yoga and which one is right for you.

The next chapter offers a general overview of 5 things you need to know before you start your class followed by chapters which cover the most common mistakes new –and experienced yogis!- make; and advice and guidance on how to get the most out of your yoga class.

The remaining chapters offer you a simple introduction into yoga philosophy and classical yoga literature, which forms the core of yoga.

As a special gift, I've included three bonuses to enhance your yogic experience.

Bonus One: Yoga In Bed: Jump-Start Your Day - Five Easy Yoga Postures You Can Do In Bed

Bonus Two: Seven Simple Seated Yoga Stretches to Get Rid Of Stress at Work

Bonus Three: Top Twelve Questions Yoga Beginners Ask About the Sun Salutation

So, let's get started and see what yoga can do for you!

How to Read This Book

There are many ways to read this book. You can pick it up and read it from front to back, put it down and say that's an interesting read.

You may be like Mary, keen to start yoga but not sure where to begin and welcome the opportunity to find out everything you can about yoga before you sign up for a class.

Perhaps you have already started yoga and would like to discover a bit more about the theory and spiritual side of yoga, as such, you will find the chapters on the history and spiritual philosophy of yoga illuminating.

Maybe you are a seasoned yogi and have a thirst for all things yoga and read anything with the word "yoga" in.

Whatever your reasons for picking up and reading I wish you well on your journey and hope this book serves you well

So let's get started with the seven most common reasons people start yoga.

Chapter 1: Seven Popular Reasons Why People Start Yoga

You cannot do yoga. Yoga is your natural state. What you can do are yoga exercises, which reveal to you where you are resisting your natural state.
Sharon Gannon

***

Have you noticed the growing trend of people who practice yoga?

There are many reasons why you may think about starting yoga. From my experience as a Sivananda yoga teacher and based on talking with students here are seven common reasons why students start yoga.

Have a look and see how many of these reasons apply to you.

1. **Yoga for Stress Relief**

A gentle yoga practice at the end of a stressful day is the ideal way to unwind and relieve tension from your body. This has to be the most popular reason why people start yoga.

Modern life is busy and full of conflicting demands. The constant hustle and bustle of your everyday life means you have a lot on your plate and often have trouble switching off and relaxing.

The essence of yoga is to encourage you to relax, take time out of your busy schedule, be present and focus on your breath. This instantly calms your mind and relaxes your body.

2. Yoga for Back Pain Relief

Have you ever suffered back pain or experienced sore, tense muscles? Yoga exercises are designed to gently stretch your muscles, increase the range of flexibility in your joints and bring suppleness to your spine. For example, yoga poses, such as the cobra, the locust or seated forward bend, all help to soothe your aching back.

3.   Yoga for Inner Peace and Calm

If you are going through an emotional crisis or recovering from a severe illness, chances are you feel unhappy and unsettled about your situation. When you feel unhappy or down, your mind is agitated and it takes longer for the body to heal. Yoga breathing exercises and meditation practices help to promote a sense of ease and calm within the body and mind which complements the healing process.

4.   Yoga for Weight Loss

Yoga is the ideal exercise to encourage you to lose weight and develop positive eating habits.

Yoga philosophy promotes a vegetarian diet based on natural, unprocessed foods. These foods tend to be wholesome and nourish your body, so you feel fuller even though you may be eating less.

Yoga teachings also encourage you to be conscious of how you eat.

Prior to eating, you bless your food and Give Thanks to the hands and souls who worked to grow your food and deliver it to your local supermarket. This sense of reverence and respect for what you eat and how you eat means you take time to select foods which nurture and nourish your body.

Instead of mindlessly snacking, eating foods on the go or slouched in front of the TV, from a yogic perspective, you consciously choose foods which nurture and nourish you. You take time to chew each morsel. In fact, there is a saying in yoga, "you drink your food and chew your drink." Meaning you take your time to fully savor and appreciate your food. The more you chew and take time to enjoy and digest your food, the deeper your sense of fulfilment from eating.

5. Yoga for Personal Development

Underpinning the physical aspects of yoga is a philosophy and way of living your life which guides you towards enlightenment. The ultimate goal of yoga is to unite with the divine and live a life of harmony, balance and inner calm.

Yoga philosophies and teachings are known as the *Yoga Sutras*. In essence the Yoga Sutras offers you a broad range of ethical and practical guidelines to living a healthy harmonious life. Many students gain inner strength, clarity and awareness of themselves through studying The Yoga Sutras. Chapters 9 and 10 give you a deeper insight into the Yoga Sutras.

6.   Yoga for Energy

Have you ever felt tired and zapped of energy?

Yoga exercises can be used to stimulate and energize your mind and body. Blocked energy is released through the chakras, which correspond to key nerve centers or plexuses in the body. As the blocked energy is released you feel energized and revitalized. More able to concentrate and, focus on the task in hand.

7.   Yoga for Health

Yoga offers you a truly holistic way of living your life. The physical postures promote a strong and healthy body, the philosophical guidelines offer you a simple way to experience life, meditation practices and breathing exercises all promote vitality and ease and comfort within your body.

As you can see, there are many reasons why you may consider practicing yoga. All reasons are valid; there is no right or wrong reason to start yoga. All you need to do is "start."

However, as Mary rightly stated, yoga is so popular how could she, a stressed, overweight, 52 year old woman, decide what sort of yoga was right for her? She hadn't exercised for years and frankly felt intimidated by the thought of wearing a tracksuit and exercising in front of a group of "skinny, flexible twenty year olds".

Mary's confidence was low and the popular image of yoga for young, white, fit women scared her. She wanted to overcome her fears yet still wasn't sure where to start or where to go. Mary did a Google search and so many classes and styles came up, that she felt even more overwhelm. They all seem to offer the same benefits, so how could she, a complete beginner distinguish between the different styles and classes on offer.

If this sounds like you, Chapter 2 "How to Choose the 'Right' Style of Yoga for You" will guide you through the maze and help you decide what type of yoga is best suited for you.

Chapter 2: How to Choose the "Right" Style of Yoga for You

Yoga teaches us to cure what need not be endured and endure what cannot be cured.

B. K. S. Iyengar

***

In this chapter, you will learn about seven of the more popular styles of yoga practiced in the West.

Once you have this information, you will discover how easy it is distinguish between the different classes on offer and choose a class that best suits your physical and emotional needs.

First we will look at the old age question: What Is Yoga?

What Is Yoga?

Yoga consists of a system of:

1. **Yoga exercises or postures, known as asanas:** Yoga poses stimulate and strengthen your "agni". Agni is your inner fire, concentrated around your solar plexus. A strong inner fire helps you to digest your food well and bring vital energy into your body.

Yoga exercises improve posture. When you are tired and lack energy, your body tends to sag; you slouch and round your shoulders. As you stretch, you release and lengthen tight back muscles and neck muscles. You feel lighter and look taller.

2. **Breathing Exercises,** known as pranayama, are designed to help you learn how to breathe correctly. In my experience of teaching, many people do not know how to breathe properly and have poor breathing habits. Yoga breathing exercises teaches you how to maximize your vitality through correct use of your respiratory system, to cleanse your body, boost your immunity and bring calmness to the nervous system and emotions.

3. **Guided Relaxation,** which promotes deep physical, mental and spiritual relaxation.

4. **Meditation and Chanting** Meditation helps to calm and focus your mind and encourages you to experience a sense of inner peace. If you are interested in meditation, ask your teacher how that is structured into the class and what type of meditation is taught. Some schools of yoga do not include chanting whereas others do.

Know you know what yoga is, the next section focuses on seven of the more popular styles practiced today.

What Are The Different Styles Of Yoga?

There are many different styles of yoga on offer. In the West, yoga classes, tend to refer to the physical aspects of yoga as opposed to the more spiritual, meditative side of yoga.

Yoga classes range from very dynamic physically challenging styles to gentle flowing restorative practices.

Hatha Yoga:

Hatha yoga is the generic term used to describe the different styles of yoga and is the most popular type practiced in the west.

The word "Hatha" is a Sanskrit word, made up of "Ha" (sun) and "tha" (moon). So, Hatha yoga literally means sun and moon joining together as one. The sun and moon represents the masculine/active (sun) and feminine/receptive (moon/lunar) principles as the opposing polarities of life. A good hatha class will be a balance of strenuous work (ha) and relaxation (tha).

Seven Popular Styles of Yoga

1. Sivananda Yoga

Founded by Swamiji Sivananda (1887–1963) this form of yoga is considered a fairly gentle to moderate pace and a good introduction into yoga.

Sivananda Yoga places emphasis on physical, mental and spiritual health. This is reflected in the class, which traditionally tends to include meditation, breathing exercises and spiritual teachings as well as the physical poses. Sivananda Yoga focuses on 12 core postures which work primarily on the spine and central nervous system.

The teachings are based on five principles for healthy living: According to Swami Vishnudevananda, if your follow these five principles you will improve your physical and mental health and deepen your spiritual connection with life. These principles are: proper exercise (asanas), proper breathing (pranayama), proper relaxation (Corpse Pose), proper diet (vegetarianism), and positive thinking and meditation.

Find out more at www.sivananda.org

2. Iyengar Yoga

B. K. S. Iyengar (b. 1918 - 1914) is the famous yoga teacher associated with this style of yoga.

In Iyengar yoga, great emphasis is placed on the structural alignment of the body. It is considered a very precise form of yoga and uses props to support the body to achieve the poses.

Iyengar yoga is considered a good introduction to yoga, especially with its strong emphasis on posture alignment, anatomy, flexibility and strength.

In my experience, an Iyengar beginners' class gives you a solid introduction into the anatomy and structure of the body as you do the poses. The use of props, which are like aids, help unfit and overweight people in particularly to feel more comfortable in the poses.

Find out more at www.bksiyengar.com

3. Ashtanga Yoga

K. Pattabhi Jois (1915–2009) is the founder of this style of yoga.

Considered a more strenuous form of yoga and definitely more physically challenging than Sivananda or Iyengar, Ashtanga yoga is very good for those who like a physical dynamic practice. It is best suited to students who are reasonable fit and in good health and in my view, looking for a workout.

Traditionally Ashtanga Yoga was taught Mysore style. This means you learnt a series of poses and practices at your own pace whilst your yoga teacher went around the room giving personal adjustments. You are normally taught the primary series and once you have mastered these poses you move onto the second, third, or fourth series. Nowadays, classes are generally led by a teacher, but traditional Mysore classes are popular.

Find out more at www.ashtanga.com

4. Bikram Yoga

Founded by Bikram Choudhury (b.1946), he introduced his system of yoga to America in 1971.

Some people refer to Bikram Yoga as "Hot Yoga" as it is taught in rooms which are heated to at least 105 degree Fahrenheit. The room is as hot as a sauna. Classes are 90 minutes long and consist of 45 minutes of standing poses and 45 minutes of floor postures. You learn 26 basic postures and two breathing exercises. As a beginner, it is essential you are in reasonable health and feel comfortable in learning yoga in a hot environment. You will sweat a lot. I like Bikram Yoga, especially during the cold winter months, as my body craves heat and the sweating helps to cleanse my body from all the extra heavy foods I eat ☺

Find out more at www.bikramyoga.com

5. Anusrara Yoga

"Anusrara" means *flowing with grace* and traditionally, students are encouraged to open to grace, surrender, and flow and connect with their heart as they practice yoga.

Founded by John Friend in 1997, Anusrara Yoga is based on alignment techniques John Friend practiced and learnt from Iyengar Yoga. Tantric philosophy and a deep sense of encouraging you to open your heart and connect with the postures as you breathe through the poses is a key feature of Anusrara Yoga.

I have yet to try an Anusrara Yoga class but friends who have, say it is a very gentle and loving experience.

Find out more about Anusara Yoga at www.anusara.com

6. Kundalini Yoga

Founded by Yoga Bhajan (1929–2004), the primary aim of Kundalini Yoga is to awaken *kundalini energy,* the energy which leads to spiritual enlightenment.

Kundalini is a very intense yoga practice. Strong breathing exercises, characterized by rapid and rhythmic exhalation, strong fast-paced asanas, mantras, mudras, (sealing gestures) chanting and meditation form the core of this active practice.

I have tried a few Kundalini Yoga classes. I like the fast deep breathing exercises, energizing effects of the asanas and chanting. It's a lovely practice especially if you feel flat and dull and need a boost of energy.

Find out more at www.yogibhajan.com

7. Baptiste Power Vinyasa Yoga

Baptiste Power Yoga is a physically challenging, flowing practice, performed in a heated room. Each class features a vigorous 90 minute vinyasa (flowing) practice designed to condition the whole body in strength, stability, flexibility and balance. Baron Baptiste founded Baptiste Power Yoga in the 1980s. The practice is physically demanding and challenging. During your practice you are encouraged to move deeper into yourself and into your own power. The idea being to prepare you, physically and emotionally, to meet the challenges you face as you transform in your daily life,

Find out more at **www.baronbaptiste.com**

As you can see, there are a variety of yoga styles to choose from.

Given the variety and range of yoga practices, I advised Mary to contact prospective yoga teachers, and ask them about the style of teaching they teach. Mary was a bit nervous about this. She was new to yoga and wasn't quite sure what questions she should ask potential teachers, plus Mary thought they might be "too busy" to answer her questions.

In my experience, most yoga teachers would be happy to answer any questions or concerns you have. You might even be offered a free trial class! So please don't feel shy in contacting teachers. Most yoga teachers have a web site, so you can make the initial contact via email.

~~~

Not Sure What Questions To Ask Your Yoga Teacher?

If you feel unsure of what questions to ask your potential yoga teacher, then the following chapter gives you a list of five main starter questions to ask before you join a new class.

Chapter 3:Five Questions to Ask Before You Join a Yoga Class

Yoga exists in the world because everything is linked.
T. K. V. Desikachar

***

As a yoga teacher, I receive many enquiries from potential students, anxious about what to expect, what they should and should not do when they join a class.

If you have these doubts and anxieties, this chapter offers you five "starter questions" you need to ask your teacher before you join a class.

1. What Are Your Qualifications?

It is always best to learn yoga from a qualified yoga teacher.

Ask your prospective teacher what style of yoga she teaches, where she trained, how long her yoga teacher's training course lasted and what subject areas where covered.

Yoga Teacher Training can be anything from a 4 week intensive while living in an Ashram (that's how I gained my Sivananda Yoga Teacher's Training Course) to 2–4 years of training, where you meet up and study with other potential teachers on a regular basis.

You can even do distance yoga teacher training courses online.

Always ask how much practical teaching experience was given on the course. Also, find out how long your prospective teacher has been personally practicing yoga, how often she practices and who inspires her to continue with her practice. To stay true to her teachings, it is essential your potential yoga teacher has her own personal practice.

2. Do You Run *Yoga For Beginners* Courses?

If you are new to yoga or looking to improve your practice it is a good idea to join a *Yoga for Beginners* Course. A beginners' class will be tailored to ensure you learn the foundations of yoga in a safe manner. Generally, Yoga for Beginners Courses is between 6 and 8 weekly sessions of 60–90 minutes each.

3. How Many People Attend Your Class?

As a beginner, look for a class that isn't too crowded—between seven to fifteen students is ideal. This allows the teacher to get to know you, observe your practice and make appropriate adjustments to your technique. A smaller class allows you to get to know your fellow yogi students and ask questions at the end of a class.

4. What Time Do You Hold Your Class And Where Do You Hold Your Class?

This is crucial. All too often students start a class without really working out how they will fit the class into their current schedule.

From experience, many people prefer to take a class on the way to or from work, or a class which is near your home. Anything too far, difficult to reach or held at an inconvenient time for you will be harder for you to start and integrate into your daily routine.

5. How Did You Get Into Yoga?

Ask your potential yoga teacher whether he has a particular niche or focus. Some teachers prefer to teach beginners whilst others focus specifically on more advanced students, children or pregnant women.

If you have any particular health needs or disabilities, this initial conversation is the ideal opportunity to see if your teacher can adapt the sessions to your needs. By talking, you will also find out more about his particular style of teaching, his overall health and wellness philosophy and any other idiosyncrasies he may have so you can gauge how comfortable you feel learning with this teacher.

Once you have this information, it becomes easier for you to find a yoga class suited to your particular health and wellness needs.

Even after asking the above questions, you may still be apprehensive and have reservations about starting yoga.

If this sounds like you, the following fifteen questions are ones which I am frequently asked by yoga beginners.

Chapter 4: Fifteen Popular Questions Asked By Beginning Yoga Students

Be patient and listen to what your body and your breath are telling you. You don't practice to be perfect, you practice to feel better. –Linda Sparrowe

***

"What is yoga?"

"What style of yoga do you teach?"

"What do I need to practice yoga?"

As a yoga teacher, I am often asked these questions by potential yoga students.

You may have heard that yoga helps you to relax, calms your mind and releases tension from sore muscles, but how can you be sure if the yoga class advertised at your local yoga studio is the right form of exercise for you?

The following is a selection of questions I am frequently asked by new yoga students.

1. What style of yoga do you teach?

This is the most popular question I am asked by yoga beginners.

There are various styles and different approaches to yoga. In essence, all yoga styles or schools practice a mixture of yoga exercises, known as asanas, breathing exercises, relaxation and in some cases meditation and chanting.

However, different schools of yoga place different emphasis on these aspects. Some yoga teachers may focus more on breathing techniques (known as pranayama), whilst another may pay more attention to the alignment of the body in the poses or body awareness and energy alignment.

Yoga classes can be taught in rooms which are heated to more than 100F (Bikram Yoga) or more traditionally, yoga classes can take place in your local health and leisure center or yoga studio. You can even have private one-on-one yoga lessons at your home.

The most common styles of yoga taught in the West are Iyengar Sivananda, Viniyoga, Ashtanga, and Bikram.

My training is in Sivananda Hatha Yoga, so my classes tend to be of a more gentle nature with emphasis on correct breathing and relaxation.

2. **What difference will yoga make to my lifestyle?**

In essence, yoga provides a framework for you to live a healthier lifestyle. Yoga practices give you tools to help you learn how to deal more effectively with stressful situations, and worrying thoughts at work and at home.

3. **I am not a vegetarian and enjoy eating meat. Can I still practice yoga?**

Yes, you can. In essence, yoga philosophy advocates a policy of non-harm, known as "ahimsa", to humans and animals. Many yogis are vegan or vegetarian, however many people who practice yoga eat meat and dairy products. The foods you eat have a major influence on your energy levels.

The following info gives you a bit more info re the influence of food on your wellbeing.

As a source of energy, food can either drain or energize you.

Many yoga practitioners believe that food contains certain qualities or "gunas".

There are three gunas: sattvic, rajasic and tamasic.

Sattvic foods are light, easy to digest, wholesome, unprocessed, and organic where possible.

Sattvic foods include seeds, fresh fruit, nuts, grains, and pulses. Sattvic foods tend to have a balancing and peaceful effect on the body.

Rajasic foods are spicy, hot, strong tasting and bitter.

This group includes foods such as strong herbs, coffee, cola, chocolate, and meat. Rajasic foods often stimulate the body.

Tamasic foods are considered dead, dull, lifeless, and stale.

They lack energy and often drain the body's energy. High-sugar cakes, biscuits, meat, pasties, and crisps are tamasic. Sattvic foods can become tamasic, such as fruit which has turned sour or gone off.

What are the best foods to eat to enhance your yoga practice?

To get the most out of your yoga practice, you ideally want to aim to eat food which provides you with maximum energy and nutrients as well as helps to repair, strengthen and protect your body from disease, e.g., raw foods, whole foods, seeds and nuts.

4. Is yoga a religion?

Yoga is multi-faceted. Yoga students come from all walks of life, social backgrounds and faiths. Yoga is not a religion, yet it offers you a philosophy and way for you to follow a healthier lifestyle. The practice of yoga, with its emphasis on cultivating inner peace and harmony, can support you to strengthen your faith.

5. What Does *Yoga* Mean?

The traditional meaning of the word *yoga* originates from the Sanskrit word 'yuj' meaning to yoke, union, join together as one. Traditionally speaking, the goal of yoga is to achieve union, connection with the Divine. In more general terms, yoga is seen as a practical way to help you achieve a state of inner balance, wholeness and calm in your life.

In the west there are many schools of yoga, but the goal is always the same, to achieve union, total harmony between body, mind and spirit traditionally in each individual and the divine.

6. What is yoga?

In today's modern (western) climate, some people view yoga purely as a form of physical exercise and place less emphasis on the deeper, more spiritual aspects of yoga. Personally, I feel it is essential you experience the physical and spiritual connection at some point in your yoga practice.

Traditionally, yoga consists of a program of stretching exercises (known as asanas) which gently open and stretch the body, increasing flexibility, suppleness and strength; breathing practices (known as pranayama) designed to cleanse the body and calm the nervous system and emotions; and guided relaxation to release body tension and promote a sense of well-being.

Some yoga classes also include meditation and chanting. Meditation helps you to calm and focus your mind and have a sense of inner peace.

7. What should I wear for a yoga class?

When you practice yoga it is essential you wear loose, not baggy, comfortable clothing. Clothes that enable you to move your body freely without restrictions and in which you feel at ease, for example, leggings, lightweight tracksuit bottoms and a cotton tee-shirt. Most yoga studios sell yoga clothing which you can try on before buying.

Some schools of yoga prefer students to wear tee-shirts which cover the shoulders and preserve modesty. In Sivananda classes, traditionally, students wear a short sleeve tee-shirt and long pants.

If practicing Bikram Yoga, it is advisable for ladies to wear a light top or sports bra and shorts. You will sweat and be uncomfortable in a tracksuit/pants and heavy tee-shirt.

Other schools of yoga, for example Iygenar Yoga, with its emphasis on the structural alignment of the body, prefer students to wear shorts above the knee so that the teacher can accurately see the body and make appropriate adjustments.

Some ladies prefer to wear leotards and leggings when they practice yoga. Make sure you wear a comfortable and supportive bra, a sports bra or well-fitted bra are ideal.

For men, I would say wear shorts or a lightweight fabric track bottom which gives you room to stretch and move comfortable. Please do not wear short shorts! Men can wear a comfortable fitted top, again available at your local yoga studio or sports shop.

Yoga is big business and the yoga clothing market huge. I always say, don't rush out and buy the latest yoga designer apparel, that is nice but at the end of the day, be practical, flexible and wear clothing which you feel comfortable in. Traditionally, yoga is not a fashion show, so bear that in mind when confronted by expensive designer clothing. It is nice but not essential.

8. Can I eat before my class?

Generally speaking, it is best to practice yoga on an empty stomach. If this is not possible, try to eat a light, easily digestible meal at least 60–90 minutes before your class.

9. I am over 40 years old, am I too old to start yoga?

Absolutely not! I have taught Chair Yoga to a group of seniors with an average age of 70 years old ☺

Yoga can be started at any age. In fact, in my experience, mature students appreciate the rejuvenating effects of yoga and approach yoga with a quiet determination to use their practice to improve their health, regain their flexibility and strength.

If you have not practiced any form of exercise for a while, then yoga, with its emphasis on gentle stretching and relaxation techniques, offers you a gentle introduction into living a more active life.

10.I am pregnant and have heard that yoga is good preparation for childbirth. Is this true?

Yes, yoga exercises and relaxation techniques are perfect preparation and exercise for pregnant women. Breathing practices and relaxation techniques help your body adapt to the physical and emotional changes your body undergoes. In addition, meditation exercises encourage you to turn your mind inwards and connect with your inner strength—all necessary preparation for labour.

If you are pregnant and this is your first experience of yoga, it is advisable to attend a Pre-Natal/Yoga for Pregnancy Class where the teacher will be able to adapt yoga poses to your particular stage of pregnancy.

11. I am really stiff and suffer from back pain. Can yoga help relieve my back pain?

If you suffer from back pain, it is essential that you seek advice from your doctor before starting any form of exercise. Yoga postures, such as the cobra and half spinal twist, can help to strengthen weak back muscles and improve the flexibility of your spine. It is important you share with your teacher the extent of damage to your spine to ensure she adapts the poses to your needs.

12. How long does a yoga session last? And what happens in a class?

Yoga is adaptable. Most classes usually last 60–90 minutes. However, when you self-practice you can practice for as little as 5–15 minutes. The main thing is to try and practice on a regular basis. Generally, your yoga class will consist of an initial relaxation, a few rounds of the Sun Salutation, breathing exercises, yoga postures and a final relaxation. Some classes include a period of guided meditation as part of the lesson.

13. I am stiff and not used to sitting cross-legged on the floor. How will I cope?

Most people in the West are not used to sitting on the floor, let alone cross-legged! If you have problems with your knees, stiff hips, or lower back pain you will find it easier to sit on a cushion or yoga block with your legs stretched out in front of you. Alternatively, you can always practice yoga seated on a chair. If you are nervous about sitting on the floor, have a quiet word with your yoga teacher before the class and she can advise you on different easy seated postures.

14. What does "asana" mean?

Asana is the term for a yoga posture or yoga pose. It literally means "steady pose."

15. What does "Namaste" mean?

"Namaste" is a sacred greeting to remember and honor the sacred, the spirit within yourself and others. When you say Namaste, you put your hands together in the prayer position in front of your heart center, bow and say "Namaste."

Now, you know the top 15 questions to ask, let's looks at some common yoga safety points you need to know about.

Like all forms of physical activity, there are dangers inherent in the activity. Although yoga is a safe, non-violent form of physical exercise, it is advisable to make sure you are aware of certain yoga protocols and safety guidelines. This will ensure you have a safe enjoyable first-time yoga experience.

The next chapter gives you an introductory guide to keeping safe when you practice.

Chapter 5: Ten Essential Practice Guidelines and Yoga Safety Tips

Just for today, offer a helping hand and caring smile to your neighbor.

Ntathu Allen

***

Yoga is a safe form of exercise. Your yoga teacher cares about you and is trained to ensure she provides a safe and happy experience for you.

However, you still have a role to play.

To maximize your enjoyment of your yoga class, it is vital you pay attention to the following practice guidelines and safety tips.

1. Treat your body with respect, care and love.

2. If you have a medical condition, always check with your doctor to make sure yoga is suitable for you.

3. Wear comfortable clothing that won't restrict your movement or get in the way when you practice the postures.

4. Never practice on a full stomach. Allow at least 90 minutes after eating before you start your class.

5. Listen to your body and move into each position slowly and carefully.

6. Practice yoga bare foot. This enhances your sensitivity of being in a pose.

7. Do not compare and compete with anyone, even yourself, in the class.

8. Focus on your breathing as you move in and out of your poses.

9. Do not hold your breath in postures. Focus on breathing slowly and smoothly through your nose as you practice. Some breathing practices, such as Alternate Nostril Breathing, encourage you to hold your breath. When the time is right, your yoga teacher will guide you through this. Some poses and sequences in Kundalini advocate exhaling through your mouth; again your yoga teacher will advise you about this.

10. Exhale as you stretch into a pose.

In practice, yoga is an ideal form of exercise to promote strength, balance and inner peace. Most yoga students are health and safety conscious, and the more you practice the easier it becomes to adopt a safe approach to your practice.

To ensure you have a safe and enjoyable yoga session, take your time and follow the above practice guidelines and safety tips.

Even if you follow the above safety guidelines, many beginners and experienced yogis still make mistakes when they practice.

To read about the five common mistakes yoga beginners make, check out the next chapter and find out what they are and how to correct these mistakes.

Chapter 6: The Five Common Mistakes Made By New Yoga Students

Trust in Spirit and allow goodness to flow into your life.
Ntathu Allen

***

To get the most from your yoga class, it is essential you avoid the five common mistakes many new students make.

Mistake #1: You Compare Yourself To Other Students.

Yoga classes attract a wide range of people with different physical abilities and emotional issues. In a class, it is tempting to compare your downward dog pose, for example, with other students doing the same pose. Generally, when you compare, you lose your focus and may even start to put yourself down or, heaven forbid, feel boastful and proud of how good you look in the downward dog pose!

Solution: Stay focused on your breath.

Yoga is a personal journey. Your yoga class is your "me time" and an opportunity to relax and let go of the constraints of work and home life. Some days your body will feel more open and flexible and you can touch your toes in the seated forward bend; on another day, you may have a stiff back and your body refuses to move into the pose. By staying focused on your breath and being aware of what is going on inside your body, you can reduce the likelihood of comparing yourself to others.

Mistake #2: You Rush Through The Poses.

It is tempting to go straight into a pose and forget to make sure your body is correctly positioned. For example, in the triangle pose you fail to make sure your feet and hips are in correct alignment and just rush straight into the pose and stretch your arm above your head. Whilst this may look correct, you run the risk of injury and do not get the full benefit of the posture.

Solution: Take your time.

All yoga poses consist of getting into the pose, being in the pose and coming out of the pose. It is essential you take your time to get into the pose, to correctly align your body, slowly breathe your way into the posture, remain there for at least 5–10 rounds of deep breathing and then slowly come out of the pose. For example, in the triangle pose, take time to make sure your feet are correctly positioned before you get into the full pose and align your hips as you move into the pose.

Mistake #3: You Get Frustrated and Annoyed With Yourself.

Most basic yoga exercises (asanas) look deceptively simple and easy to do. Consequently, a lot of new students expect to be able to go straight into the "perfect pose." However, if you have never exercised before, lead a very sedentary life or spend most of your time at a desk using a computer, your body becomes stiff and inflexible.

The expression "use it or lose it" applies to the human body. Over the years your body adapts to the demands made on it. Yoga exercises require you to stretch and move your body—although yoga is gentle, this can still be a shock to your body. You realize just how inflexible you have become over the years. I often see students get cross with themselves and moan, "I used to be able to touch my toes" as they struggle to position themselves in the forward bend pose, or have trouble raising their arms above their head as they prepare for the seated forward bend pose.

Solution: Be gentle and accept your body as it is today, not how you imagined it to be 2, 5, or even 10 years ago.

You are a living organism and, if you haven't exercised for a while, your body will be stiff and inflexible. With time, patience and regular practice, you will notice an increased range of movement and ease in your body. For example, one of my students, aged 73 years, can now place his hands just below his knees in the seated forward bend. When he first started yoga, his back and hamstrings were so stiff he reached just to his mid thighs. That is a massive increase in his range of movement and ease in his body when walking and out and about with his grandchildren.

Mistake #4: You Miss The Final Relaxation Exercise.

Most yoga classes finish with the Final Relaxation, a chance for you to lie down on your back in Savasana (the Corpse Pose) while your yoga teacher takes you through a deep guided relaxation. The Final Relaxation can last anywhere from 5 to 20 minutes. Many students who have other commitments skip the Final Relaxation and leave class early.

As a yoga teacher and yoga student, I feel the Final Relaxation is the most important yoga pose of your session. It gives the body a proper chance to fully relax, release tension and for your thoughts to turn inward and settle.

Solution: Schedule your yoga class at a time that allows you to complete the class and relax completely.

If you absolutely have to leave before the Final Relaxation, have a quiet word with your teacher at the beginning of the class and ask them to give you a quiet nod 5 – 10 minutes before you have to go, so you can have a few minutes quiet relaxation.

Mistake #5: You Think Yoga Is Just A Form Of Exercise.

Many new students do not realize that the way yoga is practiced in the West is only one path of yoga. In fact, there are four main paths of yoga practice, which all traditionally serve as a means to help you achieve your potential and unite with your divine nature:

- Karma Yoga (the path of selfless service and action)
- Jnana Yoga (the path of intellect, knowledge and wisdom)
- Bhakti Yoga (the path of devotion and love)

- Raja Yoga (the physical practice of yoga—asanas, breathing, plus spiritual, ethical guidelines, known as the Yoga Sutras or Patanjali's Eight Limbs of Yoga)

Solution: Take time to practice the four paths of yoga and study the philosophical and spiritual side of yoga, known as the Yoga Sutras.

Sign up for a yoga workshop which covers the wider psychological and philosophical aspects of yoga. Find out if your yoga studio offers Satsang, an evening of spiritual chanting, prayers, spiritual discourse and chanting. Keep your mind and eyes open to lectures on the Yoga Sutras. Visit Yoga Trade Exhibitions and Festivals and try out the different classes and workshops on offer.

Once you have got this far, you are more likely to be ready to join a yoga class.

To make your first yoga class experience even more enjoyable, turn the page and discover the seven simple steps you must take to enjoy your lesson.

Chapter 7: Seven Simple Steps to Get the Most Out Of Your First Yoga Lesson

Each morning that you arise, breathe, stretch and give thanks for the gift of yoga in your life.
Ntathu Allen

***

Yoga is a user-friendly activity. Basically, all you need is a yoga mat and comfortable clothing. Like all activities involving human interaction, to maintain a friendly and conducive atmosphere, there are certain "unspoken rules" or etiquette to yoga, which when observed helps you get more out of your yoga lesson.

1. Arrive Early

Try to be early, or at least on time, for your yoga class. Your time is precious; every second lost from your practice deprives you of the opportunity to enhance your health and nurture your body. If you arrive late, you may miss out on instructions given by your teacher or even miss out on the initial relaxation.

2. Breathe Deeply

Take time throughout your yoga practice to breathe slowly, deeply and fully through your nose. Correct yogic breathing as you practice yoga encourages healing, vibrant health and a deeper sense of wellness.

3. Maintain a Sense Of Reverence and Awe About Your Yoga Practice

Yoga is a gift you give to yourself. Take time, as you enter your class and sit on your mat, to say a few quiet words of thanks and praise for people in your life, for your breath, your health and your wealth. Yoga philosophy and teachings promote a deeper understanding of your life, purpose and goals. As you stretch your body, take time to fully appreciate the intricateness and uniqueness of your body.

4. Share a Smile or Hug With Other Yoga Students

With the threat of terrorism and economic recession, we have lost the art of gentle manners and kindness to each other. Your weekly yoga class offers you the opportunity to reconnect with other people who may be from a different culture or lifestyle. Share a smile and get to know your fellow yoga students. You may find you have more in common with each other than you would imagine. Even if you never meet your fellow yoga students outside your lesson, whilst in the class, allow yourself to be open and share your story with others. In the course of your conversation you never know whose heart you touch.

5. Enjoy Being Present In Your Body

In this age of nanoseconds and instant messaging, it is easy to get caught up in virtual time and space and forget we have a physical body and physical time scales. During your yoga lesson, take time to enjoy your body. You were born with an inner wisdom, which is stored in your body. Become body aware and tune in to see what messages you can pick up about your body.

6. Relax

Your yoga lesson is probably the only time during your week when you are actively encouraged to relax. Relaxation is vital to allow your body to heal, repair and strengthen from your daily hectic schedule. Savasana, the relaxation pose, is the most important yoga pose you can learn. Make sure you attend a yoga class where the teacher includes a minimum of 10–20 minutes Final Relaxation as part of your class.

7. Have Fun and Enjoy Your Yoga Class

Life is for living and for having fun. It is good to laugh, especially at yourself, during your yoga class. If you are not able to get into a particular pose, don't worry about it.

Smile, observe your thoughts and just do your best.

If you topple over or lose your balance in a pose, for example, in the tree pose, instead of getting frustrated and annoyed with yourself, allow yourself to topple over, laugh, and enjoy the feeling of letting go. Learn to trust your body to re-align and re-balance itself. It's all part of yoga.

What Else Do You Need To Know About Starting Yoga?

What are "yoga props"?

To further support you as you practice, there are certain yoga props you can use which make it easier for you to get into and maintain a pose.

The following chapter explains what these props are and how you use them when you practice.

Chapter 8: Seven Yoga Props to Help You Deepen Your Practice

The most important piece of equipment you need for doing yoga are your body and mind.
Rodney Lee

***

Beginner yoga students often find it difficult to get into certain poses. For example, some students have back pain and have trouble lying on their backs, or you may have tight hamstrings which makes it harder for you to get into some poses.

To support and help you work with your particular health needs and body condition, you can use a yoga prop.

Yoga props are support tools which help you get into and stay longer in a certain pose. They are also useful for students who may have tight muscles or are recovering from illness.

Here are some of the more common props or tools used in yoga.

Most yoga studios sell props. Or check out the online sites below where you can safely buy props.

Yoga Mat

Although not technically seen as yoga prop, a good-quality yoga mat is essential. Yoga mats come in a variety of sizes, styles and colors. Yoga mats can be made from organic, natural fibers which have been made with little impact on the environment, or from man-made plastic materials. Whatever style and type of mat you use make sure it has a non-slip "sticky" surface and is padded. Most yoga studios have mats for students to use at a nominal fee. But if you intend to practice regularly buying your own yoga mat is a good investment.

Yoga Relaxation Eyebags

Yoga eyebags can be made infused with lavender to promote a deeper relaxation. You simply place them over your eyes to block out light when you are laying down in relaxation pose.

Yoga Blocks

If you have tight hamstrings or a stiff back, you may find it uncomfortable to sit on the mat. To help ease and support your body you can sit on a block. This helps to lift the pelvis up and lengthen and support the back which makes it easier for you to sit cross-legged on the mat.

Yoga Strap

Straps are very useful to help you stretch that extra bit more in a challenging pose. For example in the seated forward bend you can place a strap around the soles of your feet and hold the strap as you stretch forward. Most straps are made from cotton and some straps even have a ready-made loop for your feet or hands.

Yoga Sandbag

This is an interesting prop to use. Placing a sandbag on parts of the body helps to deepen your posture.

Yoga Chair

A Yoga Chair helps students who are very inflexible, or obese, to feel more comfortable practicing yoga. When I teach Office Yoga/Yoga@Work Workshops or Senior Yoga Classes we tend to do Chair Yoga. Seated/Chair yoga enables you to participate at your own level without causing too much strain on your body. For example, you can do seated cobra whilst the rest of the class does the full yoga pose on the floor. For best results use a sturdy, straight-back chair, ideally on a non-slip surface!

Yoga Blanket

After a yoga mat, I feel a yoga blanket is the next most supportive and comfortable prop. You can fold your yoga blanket and use it under your knees if you have back pain, or under your shoulders in Shoulder Stand Pose. The best use of a yoga blanket is during the Final Relaxation, to cover yourself and keep you warm.

If you feel too unfit, stiff or uncomfortable when you practice, use a yoga prop to support you as you deepen in your yoga practice.

All these props can be bought online. Visit www.yogadirect.com or www.breatheyoga.co.uk for further details.

After practicing yoga for a while, a lot of my beginner yoga students notice that they feel differently about certain things.

Many people start yoga as a way to learn how to relax, to become more flexible and even to lose weight or heal after an emotional crisis or loss. However, over time, as they notice change in their life they are keen to discuss why this is so and express an interest in the wider spiritual and philosophical teachings of yoga.

I find this fascinating and love when students wish to go deeper into their practice.

In the following chapters we take a look at yoga philosophy, more commonly known as the Yoga

Sutras, with specific reference to the Yamas and

Niyamas.

Chapter 9: Introduction to Yoga Philosophy

The Yoga Sutras of Patanjali

From the beginning of time you respond to the calling of yoga.
Ntathu Allen

***

What are the Yoga Sutras?

The Yoga Sutras is recognized as the first complete presentation of the practical and spiritual aspects of yoga. It consists of 196 threads or commentaries which bring together all the various strands and thoughts about yoga philosophy in one main literary source. These threads cover all aspect of life, from giving guidelines on how to live a healthy industrious life right through to thoughts on how you can reach the ultimate goal of yoga - self-realization.

Who *Wrote* The *Yoga Sutras?*

Born around 300 BC, the ancient sage, Maharishi Patanjali, is recognized as key author of the Yoga Sutras. Patanjali's texts give you a set of 196 aphorisms or threads known as the Yoga Sutras. There is debate about the exact date that Patanjali wrote the sutras, but many scholars say the ancient texts are at least 2500 years old.

Tell Me More about the *Yoga Sutras*

The Yoga Sutras contains four chapters, each one covering a different aspect, or understanding of yoga. Together they offer you a road map to deepening your yoga practice. Traditionally, yoga practices were part and parcel of everyday life and these values, beliefs and ways of living are recorded in the Yoga Sutras.

- Chapter 1 talks about yoga and effects of the mind on your practice.

- Chapter 2 focuses on the Eight Limbs of Yoga.

- Chapter 3 talks about the vast potential of yoga to control and harness your mind's power,

- Chapter 4 deals with the final journey your soul makes towards "death and liberation.

What Are The Eight Limbs Of Yoga?

The Eight Limbs of Yoga is often a yoga student's first introduction into yoga philosophy.

Most yoga students, especially those in the West are aware of yoga exercises or asanas and pranayama, breathing exercises. However, did you know that asanas and pranayama are an integral part of Hatha and Raja Yoga?

Hatha Yoga refers to the physical postures and pranayama whilst Raja Yoga explores in more detail the spiritual mind-body connection. Hatha and Raja Yoga are more commonly known as the Eight Limbs of Yoga and form the second chapter of the Yoga Sutras.

The Eight Limbs of Yoga form the ethical and philosophical foundation of your yoga practice. According to the ancient sage Patanajali, in his Yoga Sutras, yoga consists of eight limbs which he called

Ashtanga Yoga. Each limb has its own identity yet still forms part of the whole system known as yoga.

The Eight Limbs or Steps of Yoga are:

1. Yama (a set of social codes for communal ethical living)
2. Niyama (guidelines for personal conduct and behavior)
3. Asana (yoga postures)
4. Pranayama (breath control)
5. Pratyahara (withdrawal and control of the senses)
6. Dharana (concentration)
7. Dhyana (meditation)
8. Samadhi (enlightenment, self-realization)

What Are The Yamas and Niyamas?

In addition, the Yamas and Niyamas are further broken down into 5 specific guidelines which give detailed explanations to guide you through your daily life.

The Yamas are:

The Yamas, deal with universal social and moral observations and sets out guidelines to encourage universal positive behaviors.

1. **Ahimsa** – Compassion and non-violence towards all beings, including animals.

2. **Satya** – truthfulness, speaking your truth in thoughts, words and behavior. Basically being honest and kind

3. **Asteya** – Non-stealing and being generous with your thoughts and actions.

4. **Brahmacharya** – Self-restraint, generally Brahmacharya refers to restraint of the sexual energy, however in its broadest sense, Brahmacharya menas self-discipline and moderation in all areas of life.

5. **Aparigraha** – Non-possessiveness and non-greed. The ability to share and to have freedom from desire. For example, not to take bribes or unasked for gifts.

The five Niyamas are:

The Niyamas are more personal observations and relate to actions which you, as an individual are encouraged to do

1. **Shauca** – Cleanliness, keeping yourself and immediate environment clean and tidy.

2. **Samtosha** – Contentment, being satisfied and accepting of your immediate situation; the ideal behind Samtosha is to allow yourself to be happy and appreciate all the blessings and tribulations in your life, yet at the same time to strive towards spiritual enlightenment.

3. **Tapas** – Relates to self-discipline; the ability to stay focused and maybe go without certain possessions in order to grow, develop and care for yourself and others, .e.g. Tapas could relate to a child giving up sweets for a period of time and giving that money instead to a local charitable cause.

4. **Svadhyaya** – Self-study and observation of your thoughts, words and actions. It includes regular spiritual discussions and studying

spiritual, philosophical literature in order to gain a richer understanding of life. It includes the ability to be reflective and introspective so that you get to know yourself on a deeper level, which helps to create clarity in your thoughts and behaviors. The more you know yourself the easier it is for you to communicate openly and honestly your desires.

5. **Ishvarapranidhana** – Refers to devotion to God. To constantly be aware of the sacredness of life and to hold reverence for all being.

As you can see the Yamas and Niyams offer you a set of highly thought of social and personal guidelines to consider as you strive to live a more harmonious and balanced life.

For more information, or classes on the Yoga Sutras, visit: http://www.flyingmountainyoga.org/
http://www.sivananda.org/
http://www.patanjalisutras.com/
http://www.discover-yoga-online.com

Chapter 10: Classical Yoga Literature

The history of yoga goes back thousands of years.

The roots of yoga can be traced back to the Indus Valley Civilization (mature period 2600–1900 BCE) that flourished in the Indus River Basin. This area covers most of Pakistan and extends into parts of modern-day India.

Several seals discovered during this period depict figures in yoga- or meditation-like postures, which suggest yoga was practiced then. As you get more into your yoga practice, you might be interested in finding out about the history of yoga as recorded in classical yoga literature. The more popular classical texts are:

The Ramaya, The Mahabharata, The Bhagavad Gita, and The Upanishads. Together; these ancient texts give you a full and detailed historical account of yoga and its origins.

Please note, the following historical literature information is extracted from a marvellous yoga resource http://www.discover-yoga-online.com

The Ramayana*

The Ramayana is an allegory for the principles of yogic living, with many 'yogic lessons' presented throughout this epic masterpiece. In essence, it is a practical yoga manual showing mankind how to live a spiritual life, with countless lessons illustrating the proper attitudes to take towards all the challenges of worldly life.

The Mahabharata

The Mahabharata is the second great yogic allegory of ancient Indian literature, written some 5000 years ago. It tells the story of the struggle of every human soul to overcome the animal passions and enable the triumph of the divine qualities of our innate, higher nature.

The Bhagavad Gita

Embedded within the Mahabharatha is most famous scripture of Indian history, the Bhagavad Gita, which itself is the ultimate textbook of yoga.

The Bhagavad Gita is comprised of eighteen chapters, each one title a specific 'yoga', a collective discourse in which Lord Krishna instructs the warrior prince Arjuna on the yogic attitude to take towards every human crisis.

Within these teachings are explanations on karma yoga (selfless action) bhakti yoga (devotion) jnaua yoga (knowledge/wisdom) and sannyasa yoga (renunciation), along with the principles of Transcendental Mind (vijnana yoga), devotional service to the Absolute (taraka-brahma yoga), the principles of meditation (dhyana yoga), and the principles of the Divine Manifestation and its extensions (vibhuti yoga).

As the most read piece of literature ever, the Bhagavad Gita takes its proper place, along with the Yoga Sutras of Patanjali, as one of the most important writings related to the science of yoga.

The Upanishads

The Upanishads (also known as the books of the vedas) also reveal this same Vedic origin of yoga.

There are numerous Upanishads, created at various times ranging from several thousand years to several hundred ago. At essence, these texts provided explanations of the mystic concepts of the Vedas in more concrete, less abstract form, and together represent the second most important repository of yogic thought.

Some of the Upanishads with particular relevance to the teachings of yoga are among the oldest, dating from the 9 to 7th century B.C., such as:

- The Katha Upanishad
- The Prasna Upanishad
- The Mundaka Upanishad
- The Chandogya Upanishad
- The Brihadaranyaka Upanishad
- The Shvetasvtara Upanishad

As you can see, when you start yoga you are entering into a timeless practice. A practice which is as popular today as it was 2000 years ago.

Where ever you are on your yoga journey, I trust this eBook offers you useful steps along your path of wholeness, health and well-being.

May you be well and live a life of peace, health and happiness.

Ntathu Allen

http://www.yogainspires.co.uk

Yoga for Beginners Unwind and De-stress at Home and at Work

Sign Up For:

As a THANK YOU for reading this book,
I WANT TO GIVE YOU A GIFT

100% Absolutely FREE

Meditation For Beginners

Learn How To Effectively Meditate In Comfort From Your Own Home! ... In 5-Minutes A Day
You just have to click...

http://freedownload5-minuteguidedmeditation.gr8.com/

Bonus 1: Kick-Start Your Day – Five Easy Yoga Exercises You Can Do In Bed

If you are too busy, too tired, and don't have the time to go to a yoga class, why not spend a few minutes each morning to practice yoga in bed?

The following five easy-to-do yoga exercises will help to mentally prepare you for the day, stretch your body and open your heart.

So, before you get out of bed, take five to ten minutes and practice this simple yoga routine.

Kick-Start Your Day - Yoga in Bed Exercises

1. As you slowly wake, gently stretch out and lie on your back. Take a few rounds of deep breathing and gradually open your eyes.

2. Slowly sit up. Make sure your back is straight and supported. Raise your arms above your head and stretch your fingers out wide. Clench

your hands, make a tight fist then stretch out your fingers.

3. Breathe in and interlink your hands. Slowly exhale as you stretch over to the right. Inhale and as you exhale return your body to the center. Inhale and on the next exhalation stretch your body to the left. Repeat this stretch twice on either side.

4. Straighten both legs on the bed and practice 10–20 "windscreen wiper" motions with your feet. Relax and take 3–5 gentle breaths.

5. Lean forward from your hips and stretch the hamstrings with one knee bent and the other leg straight. Repeat on the other leg (it you have sore knees or if this feels uncomfortable, keep both legs straight and stretch forward).

6. Hug both knees to your chest. Curl your body up into a small ball. Rock gently from side to side 5–7 times each side. Lower your head to the bed, still holding your knees to your chest, and take 3–5 deep breaths in and out. Gently move your knees from side to side, giving a gentle wringing action to the back muscles.

Lower your feet back to the bed and slowly straighten your legs on the bed.

7. After all that stretching, sit quietly for a few minutes, enjoying the stillness of your breath and the calmness of your mind.

Try and practice this simple yoga exercise sequence every day for at least a week. You will feel energized, focused, and ready to start your day.

Bonus 2: Stress Relief at Work: Seven Simple Chair Yoga Exercises to Reduce Stress

When was the last time you came home from work and felt energized, rested, and relaxed?

Or do you feel tired, tense and troubled and wonder whether you will have enough energy to cook the family evening meal, listen to your children talk about their day and make time to be with your partner?

Even if you regularly exercise, eat a balanced diet and have a supportive network of family and friends, chances are you will experience moments of overwhelm and stress during your day, especially at work where the pressure to meet tight deadlines and heavy workloads can leave you feeling stretched and stressed.

Stress at work can have a major impact on your health. The American Medical Association stated that stress was the cause of 80 to 85 percent of all human illness and disease.

Stress Statistics

Furthermore, every week 95 million Americans suffer some kind of stress-related symptom, such as high blood pressure, lower back pain, migraine, or even irritable bowel syndrome, for which they take medication.

To combat the negative effects of stress, it is vital you spend time during your day to release the build-up of stress chemicals in your body. Once they're released you feel better, more alert and able to concentrate on the task at end.

The following seven easy yoga stretches can be slipped into your day to help release stress and tension in your body and to calm your mind.

1. **Feet and Ankles Stretch** – Sit comfortably on your chair with a straight back. Stretch your legs out and slowly rotate your ankles and feet five times in each direction.

2. **Seated Spinal Twist** – Sitting on your chair, cross your left leg over your right leg. Place your right hand on your crossed knee. Keeping your back straight, slowly turn your body to the left and look over your shoulder. Gently release and turn back to the center. Change legs and twist the other way.

3. **Seated Forward Bend** – Sitting on your chair, feet firmly placed on the floor, breathe in. As you breathe out, slowly bend your upper body forward toward the ground like a rag doll. Relax and take 3–5 deep breathes before slowly returning to an upright position.

4. **Seated Cobra/Backward Bend** – Sit comfortably on the edge of your chair. Make sure your feet are facing forward and resting squarely on the floor. Rest your palms on your thighs. Breathe in. As you breathe out, gently lift your chest, lower your head back and arch backwards. Breathe deeply and relax. Slowly return your body to center.

5. **Stretch Arms Above Your Head** – Sitting or standing, raise both arms above your head and

stretch out through your fingers. Hold your left wrist with your right hand and gently stretch over to your right. Relax and breathe into the stretch. Return to the center. Switch arms and repeat on the other side.

6. **Neck Stretch** – Sitting tall and straight, rest your hands on your lap. Breathe in. As you breathe out slowly lower your right ear to your right shoulder. Ease into the stretch and gently return your head to center. Repeat on the other side.

7. **Chewing Gum** – Pretend to chew a large piece of chewing gum. Chew, chew, chew. Close your eyes and gently massage your cheeks, forehead, temples, and head with your fingers.

Choose any two or three of the above yoga stretches and practice them throughout your day. You will soon feel calmer and more able to survive stress at work.

Bonus 3: Top Twelve Questions Yoga Beginners Ask

About the Sun Salutation

Every morning, when you arise, breathe, stretch and energise your mind, body and soul.

***

Once you join a yoga class, you may notice that at the start of most yoga lessons your teacher leads you through a yoga sequence known as the Sun Salutation.

Most schools of yoga have their own version of the Sun Salutation. Here are 12 popular questions I am asked about the Sun Salutation.

1. **What is the Sun Salutation?**

The Sun Salutation is an ancient yoga practice that draws energy and sunlight into the mind and body. It is made up of 12 different movements or positions which form a graceful sequence.

2. What part of the body does it stretch the most?

The Sun Salutation limbers up the whole body and mind. Each of the 12 positions stretches the spine in different ways, thus giving movement to the whole spinal column and greater flexibility to the limbs.

3. Why is it always practiced at the beginning of a yoga session?

The Sun Salutation helps to limber up the body which makes it easier for you to do the rest of your session. It also helps to focus your mind for the session ahead.

4. How quickly am I supposed to do the Sun Salutation?

Generally speaking, the Sun Salutation is performed gracefully and in time with the movement of the flow of your breath. It is designed to be a smooth, fluid sequence which harmonizes the mind and body. The main thing is to be aware and connected with your breath.

5. Why is it called the Sun Salutation?

The correct Sanskrit name for the Sun Salutation is Surya Namaskar, which means Salute to the Sun. Its origins lie in a worship of Surya, the Hindu solar deity. In ancient times, the sun was considered to be the deity for health and long life. Traditionally, you would practice the Sun Salutation as a dance to the sun at dawn break as part of your spiritual practice. In honoring the sun, you would bring sunlight and energy into your body.

6. What are the main physical benefits of practicing the Sun Salutation?

The main physical benefit is it brings flexibility to the body, particularly the spine. It also helps to regulate the breathing, and helps to distribute blood and energy to all the organs, as circulation is stimulated.

7. What are the other benefits?

Spiritually, practicing the Sun Salutation realigns and centers your core. It brings focus to the mind. Traditionally, each position is associated with a particular mantra.

8. How long is one round?

A full round of Sun Salutation is considered to be two sets of the 12 poses, leading first with the right leg and then with the left leg.

9. How many round am I supposed to do at a time?

Traditionally, yogis practiced 12 rounds in honor of the 12 names of the sun according to the monthly sign of the zodiac. As a beginner, it is advised to practice 3–5 rounds until you feel comfortable doing more.

10. Does it matter which way I face to do the Sun Salutation?

Traditionally, the Sun Salutation is always practiced facing in the direction of the rising or setting sun.

11. I'm too stiff/use a wheelchair; can I still do the Sun Salutation?

Yes, you can. Ask your yoga teacher to show you how to do the seated Sun Salutation. Alternatively, check out Nischala Joy Devi in *The Healing Path of Yoga,* Three Rivers Press, 2000. Nischala offers very good seated Sun Salutation and a standing version with a chair.

12. Can I practice the Sun Salutation at home by myself?

Definitely. Once you feel confident and comfortable with the sequence, daily practice of the Sun Salutation forms an ideal Home Yoga Practice.

Get Even More

As a THANK YOU for reading this book, I want to give you a GIFT

you a GIFT

100% Absolutely FREE

Meditation For Beginners

Learn How To Effectively Meditate In Comfort

From Your Own Home!... In 5-Minutes A Day!

You just have to click...

http://freedownload5-minuteguidedmeditation.gr8.com/

Special Request – Customer Reviews

Thank you for taking the time to read this book.

If you enjoyed reading it, would you please pop over to Amazon and leave a review because it helps other readers make an informed decision about what books to read. Also, as a self-published author, it helps to build up my profile and encourages me to keep on writing. Thank you!

To leave a short review and a 5-star rating on Amazon (if you think I deserve it!), simple click on "Write a Review", enter a title for the review, for example "Great Read" and write a few short sentences explaining what you like about the book and why you would recommend it (hopefully you'll recommend it!). And that's it.

Thank you. And finally, you can check out other books I've written over on my Amazon Central Authors page, which you can visit when you click here

http://amzn.to/1d4uC9D

Please leave us a short review and 5-star rating on Amazon (if you think we deserve it)!

About The Author

Ntathu Allen

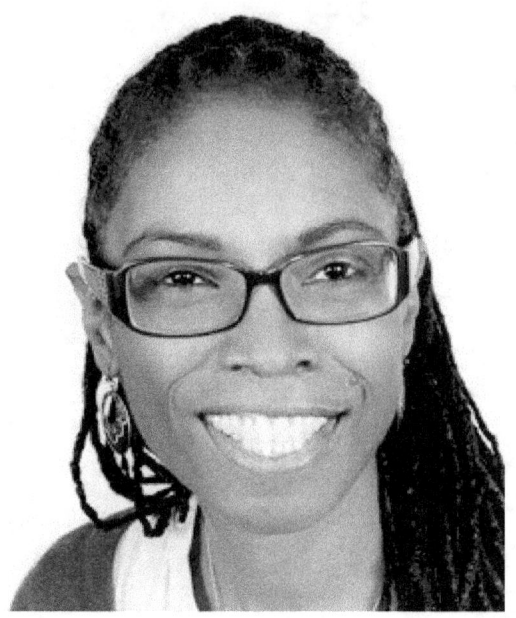

Ntathu Allen is a yoga teacher, who specializes in the areas of yoga for stress relief, inner peace and calm

Ntathu has lovingly combined her personal spiritual practices, professional yoga and meditation training and therapeutic bodywork skills to develop **Yoga Inspires**. She first got into yoga when pregnant with her eldest daughter, who is now 24 years. Ntathu's midwife advised her to "learn how to relax" as she was stressed and always tired from working, at that time, as a Probation Officer, in a challenging inner city borough of London. However the demands of looking after her young family (3 daughters) and work commitments, especially supervising vulnerable young offenders and supporting their families, were too stressful and took its toll on her health and time spent at home with my family. In 2003, Ntathu travelled to India to train as a Sivannada Yoga Teacher and in 2004 resigned from the Probation Service to set up her own yoga, meditation and wellness business.

Ntathu now teaches overworked and stressed-out professional and business women, who want to live a calm, healthy and abundant life, learn how to relax, reduce stress and make time for yourself – so you can stop rushing around and feeling overwhelmed; which means you enjoy a more positive, productive and peaceful day (even if you are swamped with work!) She shares her extensive knowledge of yoga through her inspirational and spiritual range of ezine articles, blogs and Kindle eBooks and offers private Hatha yoga and guided meditation lessons as well as corporate and community based classes and workshops. Ntathu believes that taking time out of your busy schedule to relax, reduce stress and reenergize helps you have a positive, productive and peaceful day. For more information on Ntathu's inspirational range, visit www.yogainspires.co.uk , join the free Yoga Inspires loving community, and start to reduce stress and feel calm and peaceful now!

You can also connect with Ntathu on…

Twitter: http://twitter.com/yogainspiresyou

Blog: http://yogainspires.co.uk

Facebook: http://www.facebook.com/yogainspires

LinkedIn: http://www.linkedin.com/groups/Yoga-Inspires-Life-One-Breath-3702115

Ezine Articles:
http://ezinearticles.com/?expert=Ntathu_Allen

Feel free to send Ntathu any questions you may have on yoga!

ntathu@yogainspires.co.uk

Check Out My Other Books

Below you'll find some of my other books that are popular on Amazon and Kindle. Simply click on the links below to check them out. Alternatively, you can visit my author page on Amazon to see other work done by me.

Back Care – Yoga Exercises for Lower Back Care at Work: Reduce Stress, Boost Energy and Improve Posture http://amzn.to/1jXOY9r

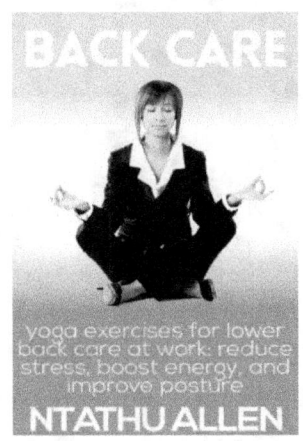

Yoga For Beginners – How to Choose Your First Yoga Lessonhttp://amzn.to/1IPb6Q2

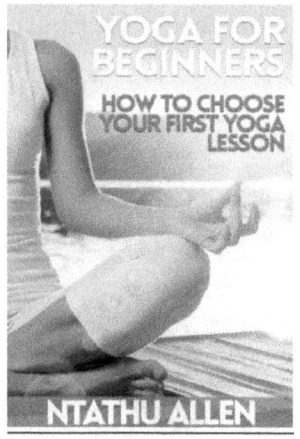

Yoga For Beginners – The Busy Woman's Guide to Easy Yoga Poses and Meditation Techniques to Relieve Stress at Work and Find Peace and Quiet at Home

http://amzn.to/1mzNt13

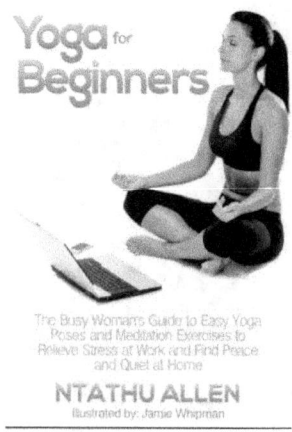

Healing After Loss – Devotional Poems for Healing and Peacehttp://amzn.to/1nQPVQk

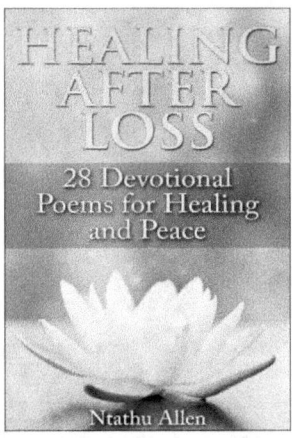

Pray As You Go: Seven Meditation Techniques You Wish You Knew for Healing andHappinesshttp://tinyurl.com/l73sodq

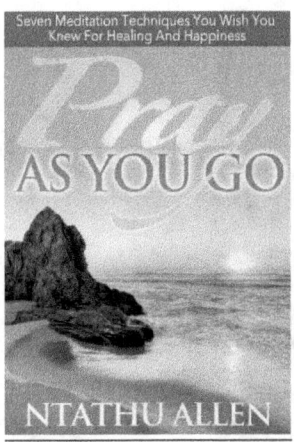

Work Happy: 26 Empowering Tips for Women Entrepreneurs to Stop Stress Now, Supercharge Your

Energy and Finally Enjoy Work

http://tinyurl.com/pgb6jkp

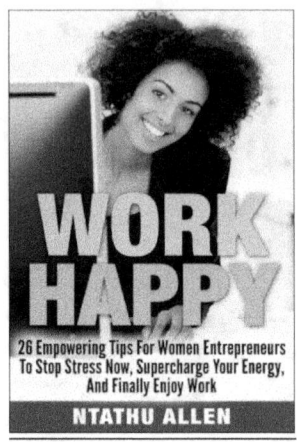

Quick Fix Meditation: The Ultimate Meditation Guide for People Too Busy to Meditate

http://www.amazon.com/dp/B00PE8SYTW

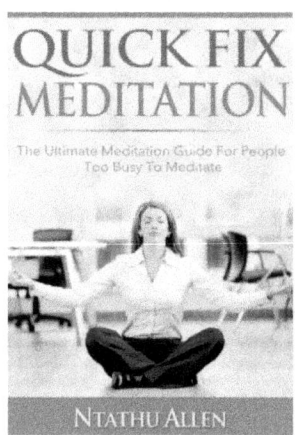

If the links do not work for whatever reason, you can simply search for these titles on the Amazon website to find them

Enjoy this book?

Please leave a review below, and let us know what you liked about this book by clicking on the Amazon image below,

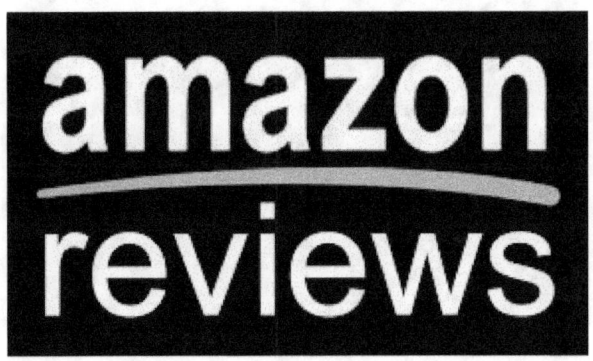

and click on Digital Orders.

The above link directs to Amazon.com. Please change the .com to your own